The Visual Guide to Asperger's Syndrome and Anxiety

by Alis Rowe

Also by Alis Rowe

One Lonely Mind
978-0-9562693-0-0

The Girl with the Curly Hair - Asperger's and Me
978-0-9562693-2-4

The 1st Comic Book
978-0-9562693-1-7

The 2nd Comic Book
978-0-95626934-8

The 3rd Comic Book
978-0-9562693-3-1

Websites:
www.alisrowe.co.uk
www.thegirlwiththecurlyhair.co.uk
www.womensweightlifting.co.uk

Social Media:
www.facebook.com/thegirlwiththecurlyhair
www.twitter.com/curlyhairedalis

The Visual Guide to Asperger's Syndrome and Anxiety

by Alis Rowe

**Lonely Mind Books
London**

First published in 2014
by Lonely Mind Books
London

Copyright © Alis Rowe 2014

All rights reserved. No part of this publication may be reproduced in any material form (including photocopying or storing it in any medium by electronic means and whether or not transiently or incidentally to some other use of this publication) without written permission of the copyright owner except in accordance with the provisions of the Copyright, Designs and Patents Act 1988 or under the terms of a licence issued by the Copyright Licensing Agency Ltd, 90 Tottenham Court Road, London, England W1T 4LP. Applications for the copyright owner's written permission to reproduce any part of this publication should be addressed to the publisher.

Warning: The doing of an unauthorised act in relation to a copyright work may result in both a civil claim for damages and criminal prosecution.

Printed and bound in the USA

For people with Asperger's Syndrome and their Neurotypical families and friends

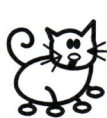

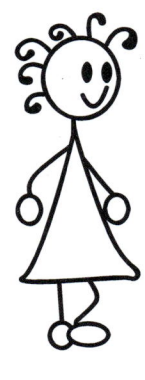

hello

This book is all about anxiety in people with Asperger's Syndrome and autism spectrum disorders (ASD).

A lot of people think anxiety is the same for everyone, but I think anxiety in people with ASD has different reasons and causes, and consequently it needs to be managed differently.

I hope you enjoy this book.

Alis aka The Girl with the Curly Hair

Contents

p11   **What is anxiety?**
p19   **Anxiety and ASD**
p39   **Strategies for living with anxiety**
p55   **Strategies for communicating about anxiety**
p69   **Strategies for anxiety in social environments**

What is Anxiety?

For people with ASD, anxiety usually stems from experiencing life as a series of random events

The person remains in a heightened state of tension and alertness, not knowing what might happen next

Anxiety is actually a natural response caused by the 'fight or flight' hormone. The problem is when the anxiety is so high that it becomes debilitating, as is often the case in the person with ASD

There are some situations that make everybody anxious, for example:

	Neurotypical anxiety	ASD anxiety
Taking an exam	High	Higher
Going to the doctor	High	Higher
Acting in a play	High	Higher
Going on a first date	High	Higher

But note this. Everyone experiences a resting level of anxiety and a higher level of anxiety during stress. However, typically, at rest the anxiety of the NT will be very low. The person with ASD at rest may experience similar anxiety to a stressed NT

Comparison of ASD/NT anxiety levels:

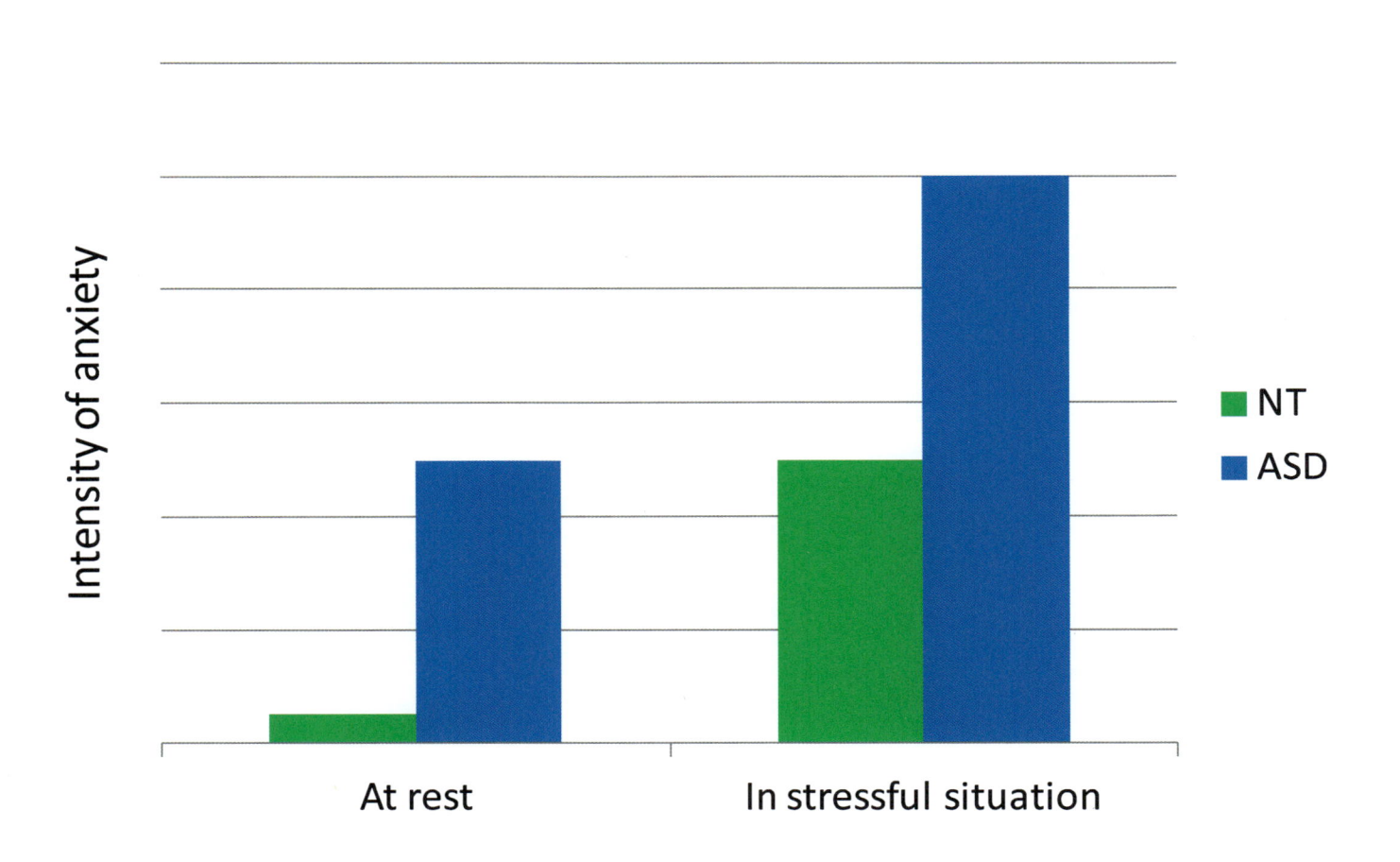

Intensity of anxiety

| | At rest | In stressful situation |

- NT (green)
- ASD (blue)

For most people, anxiety begins – or worsens – at adolescence

Child:
Parents are largely responsible for their child's routines and friendships;
Primary school is generally small and safe;
Teachers look after them

Adolescent:
They become aware they are 'on their own' socially;
Increased awareness of self;
Friendships become their own responsibility rather than their parents;
Secondary school is larger, complicated and variable;
Internal and external body changes

Adult:
High self-awareness;
Pressure to act their age – jobs, money, university, family, partners, etc.;
Without the structure of school, it can be hard to sustain friendships

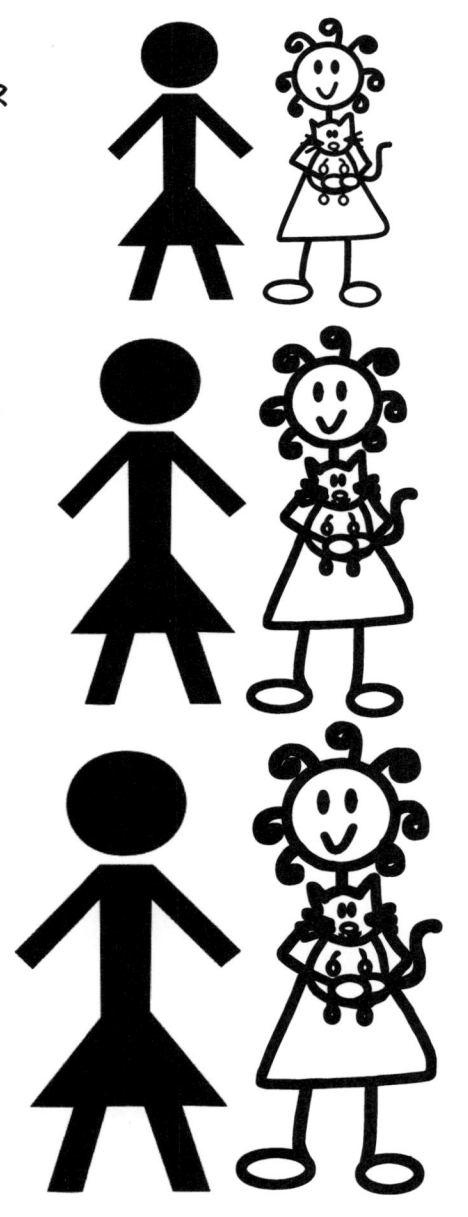

Anxiety and ASD

People on the autism spectrum may have two main triggers for anxiety:

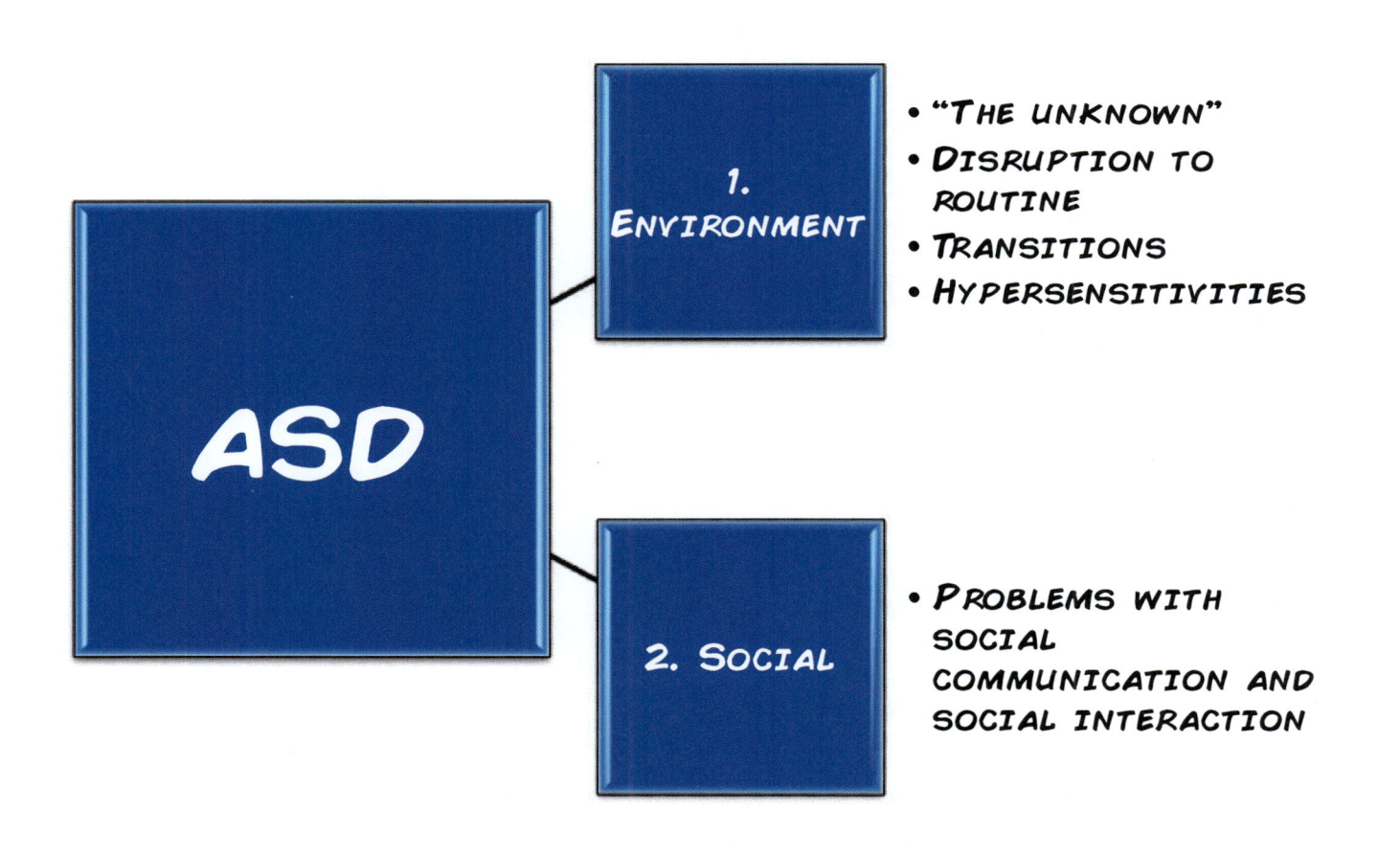

ASD

1. Environment
- "The unknown"
- Disruption to routine
- Transitions
- Hypersensitivities

2. Social
- Problems with social communication and social interaction

By the way, 'social anxiety' and **Asperger's Syndrome (or ASD)** are not the same thing

There may be however, an overlap of symptoms

Social anxiety vs. ASD anxiety

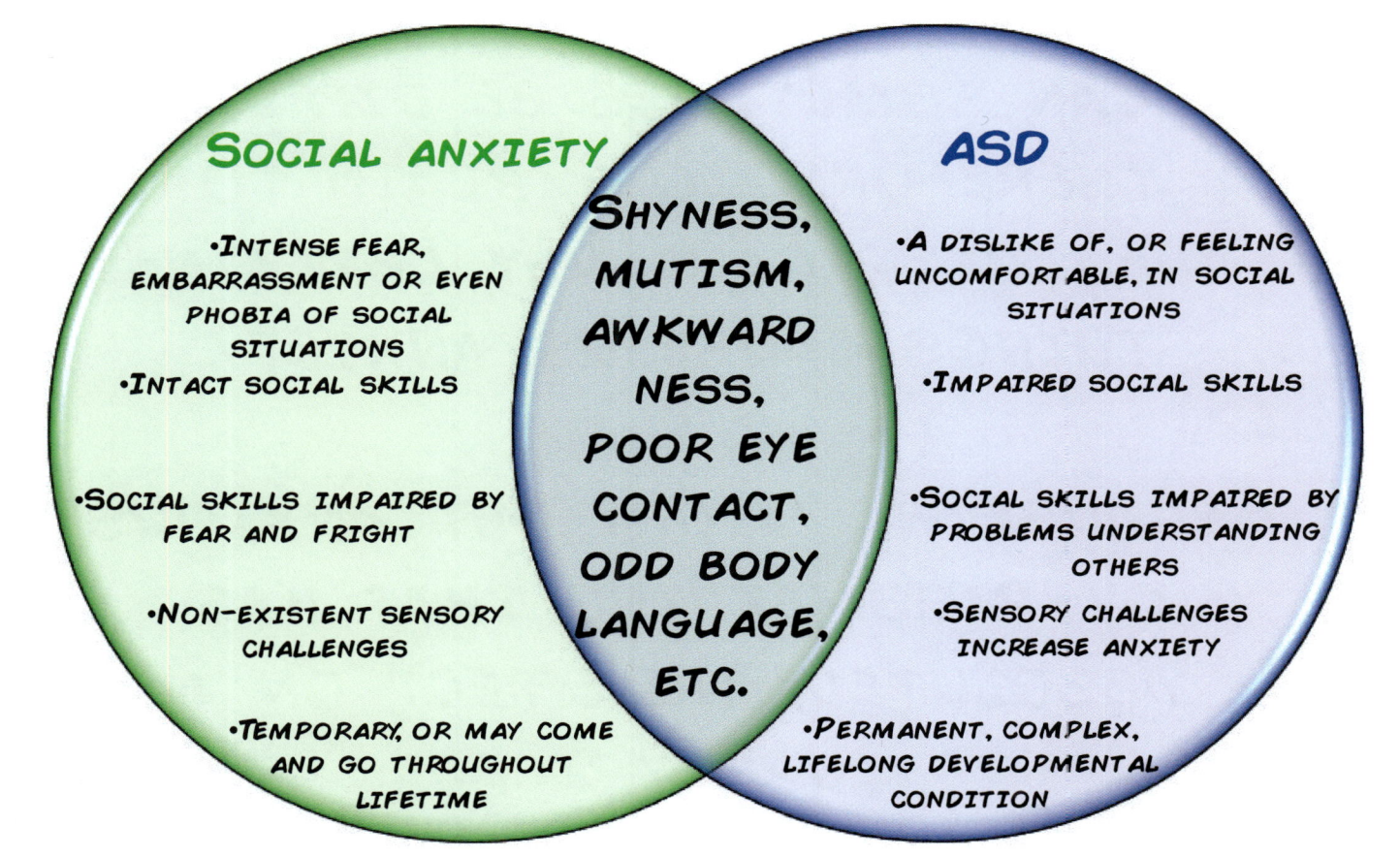

Social anxiety

- Intense fear, embarrassment or even phobia of social situations
- Intact social skills
- Social skills impaired by fear and fright
- Non-existent sensory challenges
- Temporary, or may come and go throughout lifetime

Shared
Shyness, mutism, awkwardness, poor eye contact, odd body language, etc.

ASD

- A dislike of, or feeling uncomfortable, in social situations
- Impaired social skills
- Social skills impaired by problems understanding others
- Sensory challenges increase anxiety
- Permanent, complex, lifelong developmental condition

Because **people with ASD** see the world differently, it means they react to things differently too

It can sometimes be difficult therefore, to explain to **neurotypicals** why certain things cause us anxiety

Because we might get anxious over something that has absolutely no effect on a **neurotypical**

Many people experience social anxiety without having ASD

Many people with ASD experience anxiety in social situations… as a consequence of their condition

See next page…

In DSM-5*, ASD is diagnosed using two domains:

1. restricted, repetitive patterns of behaviour, interests or activities (environment),

and

2. Social communication and interaction (social)

*The Diagnostic and Statistical Manual of Mental Disorders, Fifth Edition

Anxiety is the consequence...

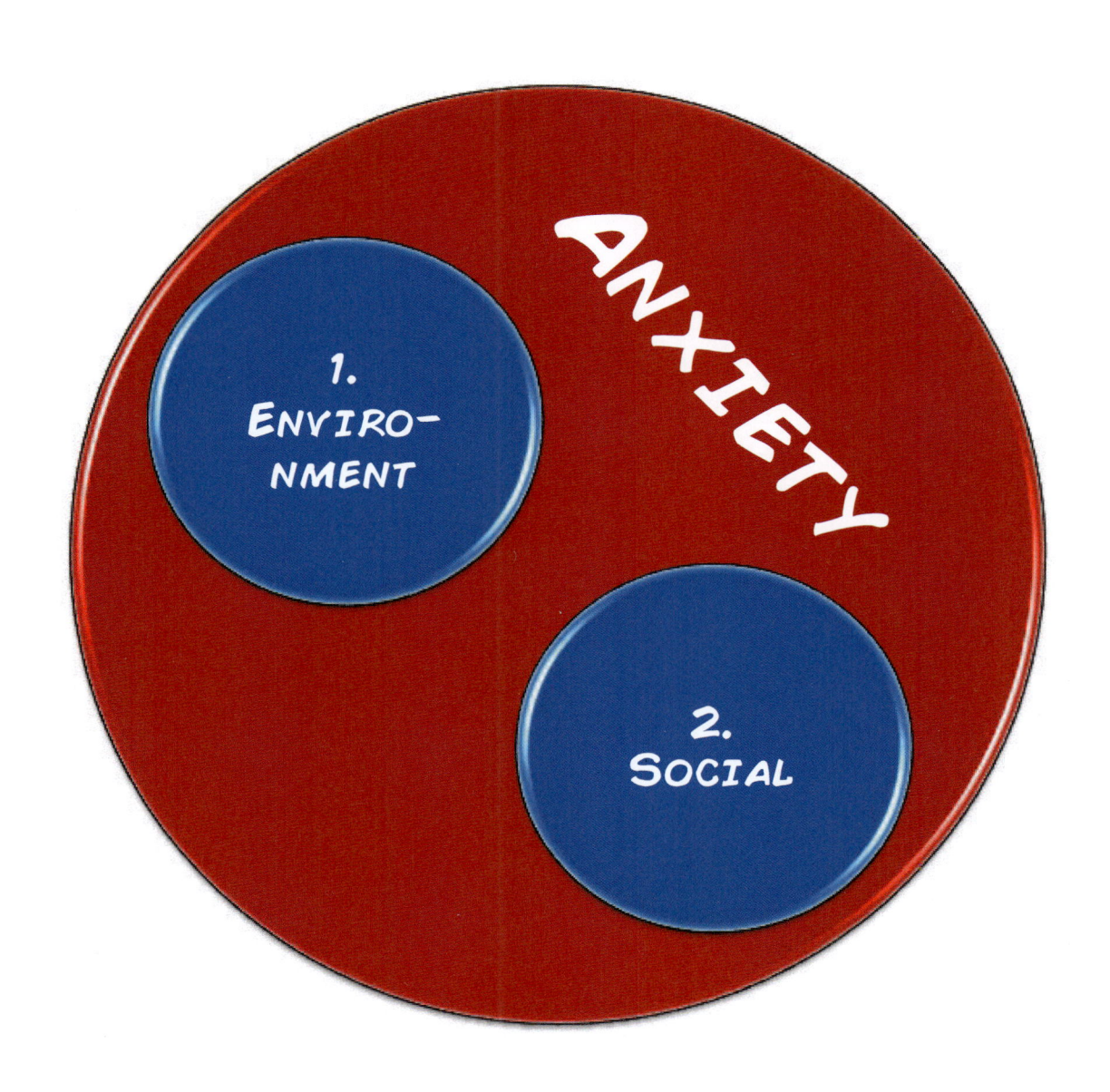

ANXIETY

1. Environment
2. Social

So why do these two things ('Environment' + 'Social') cause anxiety?

ASD may cause sensory behaviours, which may cause anxiety...

- We can be hyper-sensitive to noise/touch/light and feel constantly 'on alert' in new environments and situations. Being over-sensitive can be very disorientating

- We may have sensory issues regarding our diet, e.g. colours, textures, flavours etc. All these can make someone become very anxious about new situations when we are expected to eat

- Our parents may know our triggers and be able to help and reassure us but when they are not there, we have to manage on our own

- Sometimes we can't even go outside, for fear of being in a crowd, such as when we go shopping

- 'Normal' sounds such as alarms, door bells, Hoovers, lawn mowers and even background sounds from the TV can overwhelm or distract us

- Cold, rainy, windy and stormy weather can be disorientating and unsettling

- Certain loud or sudden sounds can be frightening

ASD MAY CAUSE A NEED FOR ROUTINE AND STRUCTURE, WHICH MAY CAUSE ANXIETY...

- We need to know what is happening next, how long it will last, where we will have to go, etc. It's not always possible to get this information

- We like doing the same things and when things change or get interrupted, that upsets us

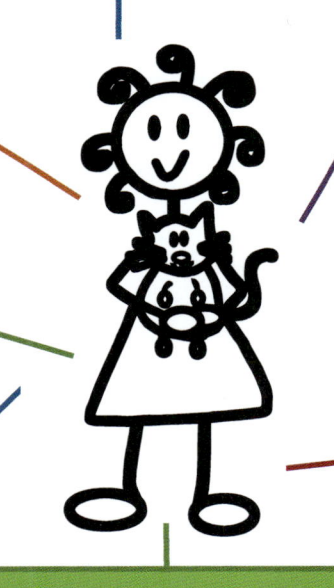

- Start and end times are important to know, but a lot of things only give the start time

- Unlimited free time can be horrible if we lack the intuition needed to occupy ourselves

- The world is very unpredictable and spontaneous, which is very hard for those of us who naturally crave the opposite

- Unexpected changes in routine, timetables, the people we work with, food, clothing etc. can all cause anxiety

- We do not understand others very well. Having structure to social situations allows us to understand others a lot better than without it

ASD MAY CAUSE DIFFICULTIES WITH SOCIAL COMMUNICATION WHICH MAY CAUSE ANXIETY...

- Where do I look when I am speaking to someone? It feels awkward to keep looking in their eyes. It's hard having them look into mine

- I can't work out when somebody might be bored with what I am saying and when I should change the topic

- I don't know how close to stand when I am talking to someone. I always worry I might be too close so I consciously make an effort to move further away

- How do I end a conversation without seeming rude?

- When is it my turn to speak? When is it their turn to speak? How long do I pause for?

- Why did they say they were only going to be "5 minutes?" It's been 11 minutes and they're still not back

- What does it mean when they wink at me, or when they pat my back?

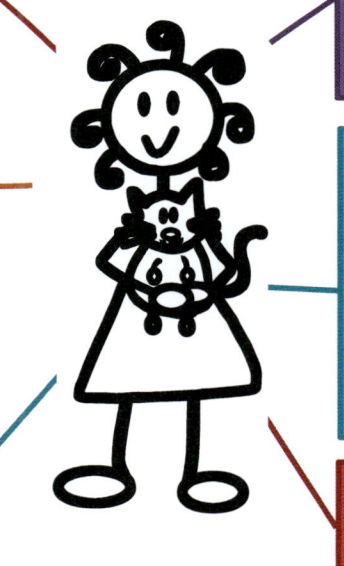

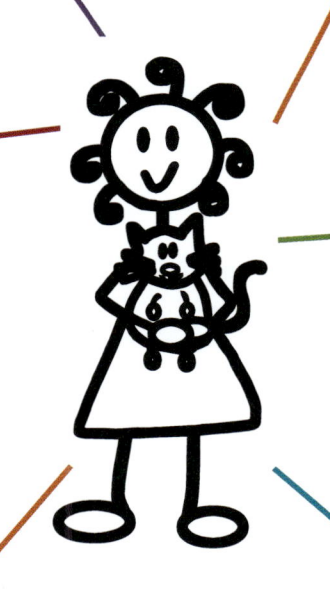

ASD MAY CAUSE DIFFICULTIES WITH SOCIAL IMAGINATION WHICH MAY CAUSE ANXIETY...

- We always have salmon on Mondays. But today is Monday and we don't have any salmon in the fridge. Does this mean I wont have any dinner tonight?

- I don't understand why Mum is upset with me. She is sick in bed. I brought her medicine. What more does she want me to do?

- I don't know what to do when Dad shouts at me and says "The house is a mess." Which bit is a mess? What exactly does he want me to do?

- Why does my partner want me to kiss and hug him every morning before he goes to work? Why does he feel unloved if I don't do it?

- My friend's husband had an affair and she asked him to leave the house and go and live somewhere else. Now she says she feels abandoned. But she asked him to leave. I don't understand why she feels this way

- Me and my friend have always cycled round the same park. Now she wants to cycle in a different park. I don't want to

ASD MAY CAUSE DIFFICULTIES WITH SOCIAL INTERACTION WHICH MAY CAUSE ANXIETY...

- I find it really hard to talk to people. Most of the time, I just stay on own and will only speak when spoken to – and even then sometimes I am silent

- I don't feel like I can be myself when I am in public. When I make an effort to look nice, smile and chat to everybody about the weather and what's on the T.V., I feel like I am not being me

- Everybody else hangs out together at the evenings and weekends. But I'm really tired by then and need to be on my own. I feel different

- I feel like I can't go to my friend's birthday party because it's at the 'wrong' time with the 'wrong' food

- I like to wear the same clothes every day. I don't really like showering or combing my hair. I don't care about brands or labels and I don't wear makeup. I look different

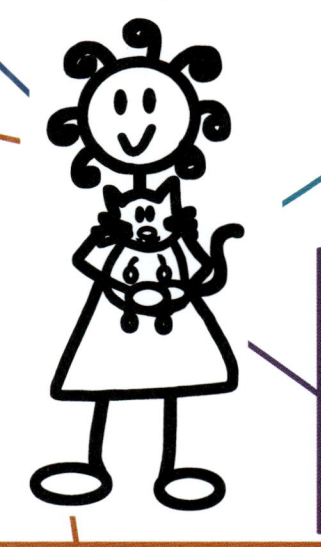

- Lots of people get excited about going on holiday or going clubbing. I don't enjoy those things. I feel different

- Why does everyone else seem to really enjoy pairing up or working in groups? I just get left out

Strategies for living with anxiety

Have a routine

If things are predictable, the person with ASD will feel much more secure and a lot less anxious...

Use a daily timetable

Timetables create structure and routine which take away uncertainty and help to make daily life more predictable

7am	8am	9am	10am	11am	12pm	1pm	2pm	3pm	4pm
Walk the dog	Breakfast	Work	Work	Work	Lunch	Work	Work	Work	Gym

Mark off the days

Cross off the days as they pass so that the person can see how close they are getting to a particularly anxiety-provoking event, such as a holiday

1st	2nd	3rd	4th	5th	6th	7th	8th	9th
X	X	X	X	X	X	X	X	Holiday

Note: For some people however, the countdown is more anxiety-provoking than being given very short notice

Schedule smartly

If we schedule the most anxiety-provoking task to take place at the beginning of our day, it can reduce the time spent worrying

For example, an event at 8am means only two periods of anxiety compared to eight periods of anxiety if the same event were scheduled for 2pm:

The night before	7am	8am	9am
Anxiety	Anxiety	Anxiety-provoking event	Recovery

The night before	7am	8am	9am	10am	11am	12pm	1pm	2pm	3pm
Anxiety	Anxiety	Anxiety	Anxiety	Anxiety	Anxiety	Anxiety	Anxiety	Anxiety-provoking event	Recovery

Use visual timetables

Many people with ASD process visual information better than verbal or written information. We can create visual timetables on pieces of paper, on the fridge or with stickers

For example, our nightly routine might look like this and is displayed on the bedroom wall:

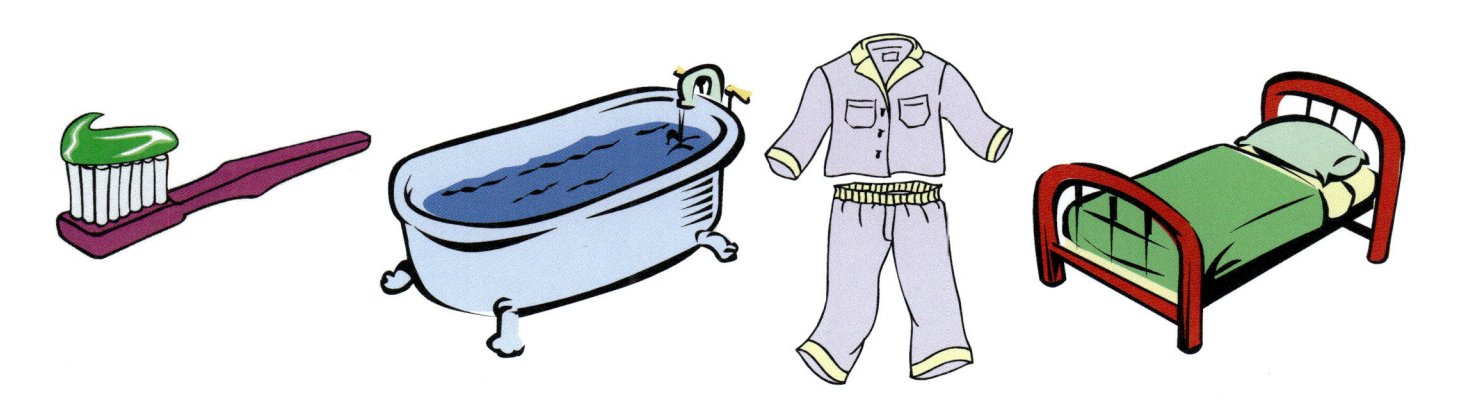

Know start and end time

Find out when a meeting, task or activity, etc. is going to end. It is common to know when something is going to start, but knowing when it's going to finish is just as important

Either we can ask for the expected duration or specify an end time ourselves

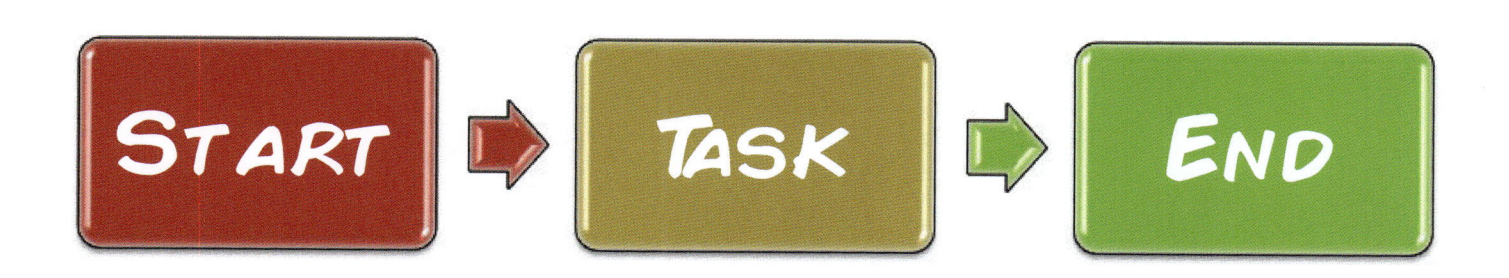

Start ➡ **Task** ➡ **End**

Show when it's time to stop

Timers can help the person "see" the rate of the passing of time

Physically cross it off on the calendar or timetable

Use a Stop sign

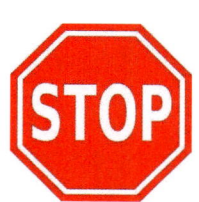

Write the expected end time on a piece of paper or on a white board

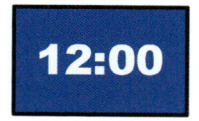

Write 'finish'

Cover over the work with a piece of blank paper (or turn to a new, blank page)

Manage Transitions

Change is difficult for people with ASD, not just the bigger picture changes such as going to a new school or moving house, but smaller changes such as moving from one activity to another, i.e. from A to B

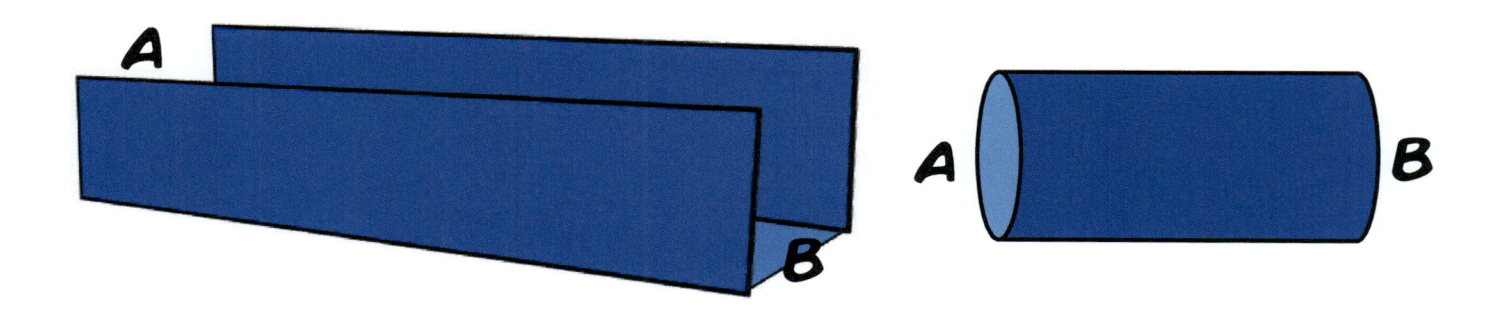

Go through hallways and corridors... or play tunnels

Strategies for communicating about anxiety

Learn to recognise anxiety

People with ASD may not even know what anxiety is so it's helpful to talk to our loved ones and have them teach us the physical signs to recognise. We can draw an outline of our body and write down some signs:

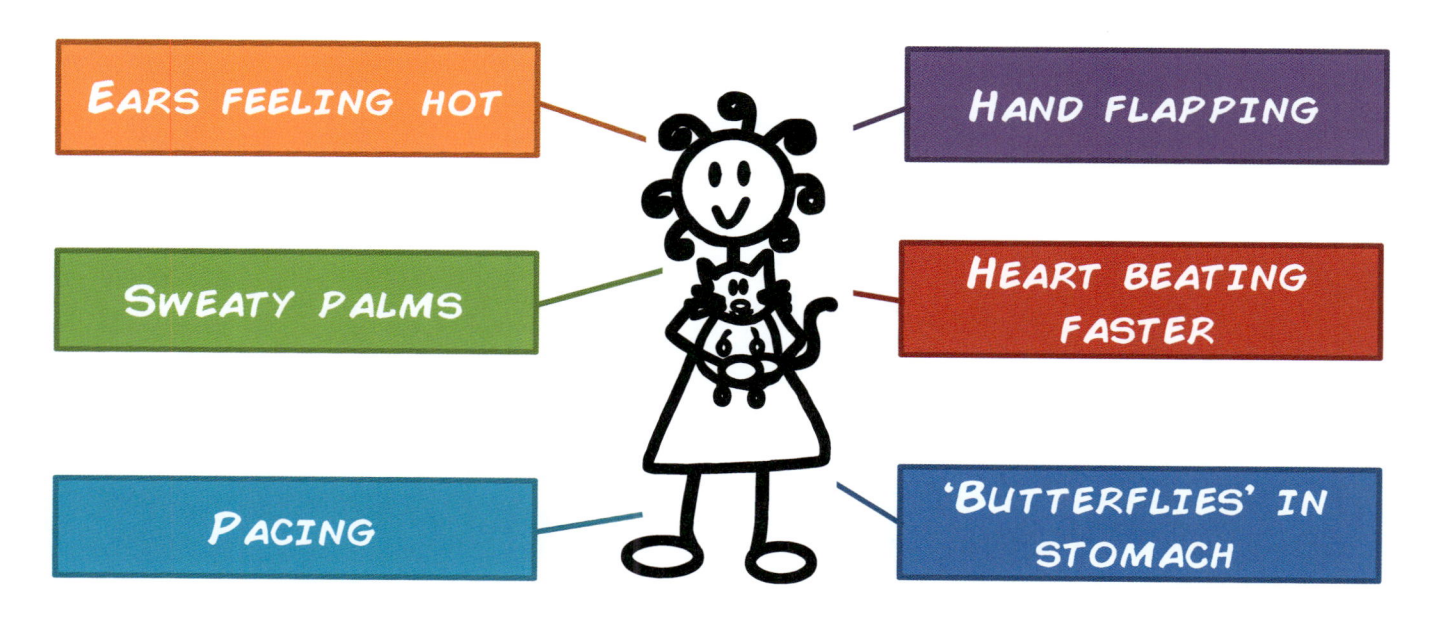

- Ears feeling hot
- Sweaty palms
- Pacing
- Hand flapping
- Heart beating faster
- 'Butterflies' in stomach

Use an anxiety number scale

People with ASD don't always find it easy to express their emotions, or tell people how they are feeling. Use a scale to communicate anxiety levels before meltdown occurs

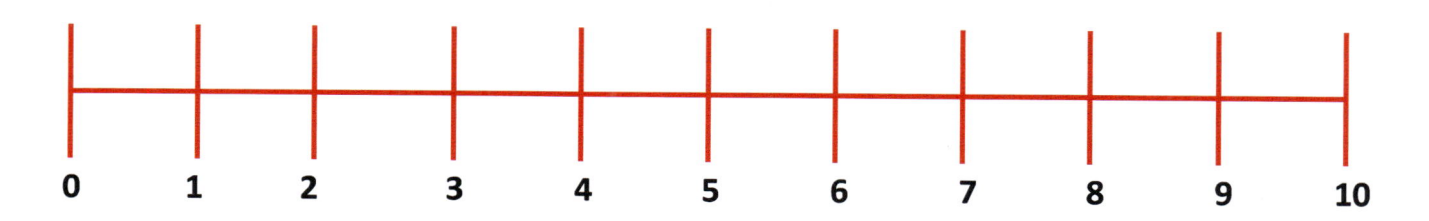

0 1 2 3 4 5 6 7 8 9 10

Agree on a number when another person needs to intervene to prevent meltdown. **The person with ASD** can also learn to take themselves away to calm down when they feel their anxiety rising

0 = very happy/relaxed
10 = very unhappy/anxious

Recognise triggers

The person with ASD needs to first know what their personal triggers are before they can take measures to manage them

Once we know what they are, it is easier for us develop coping strategies

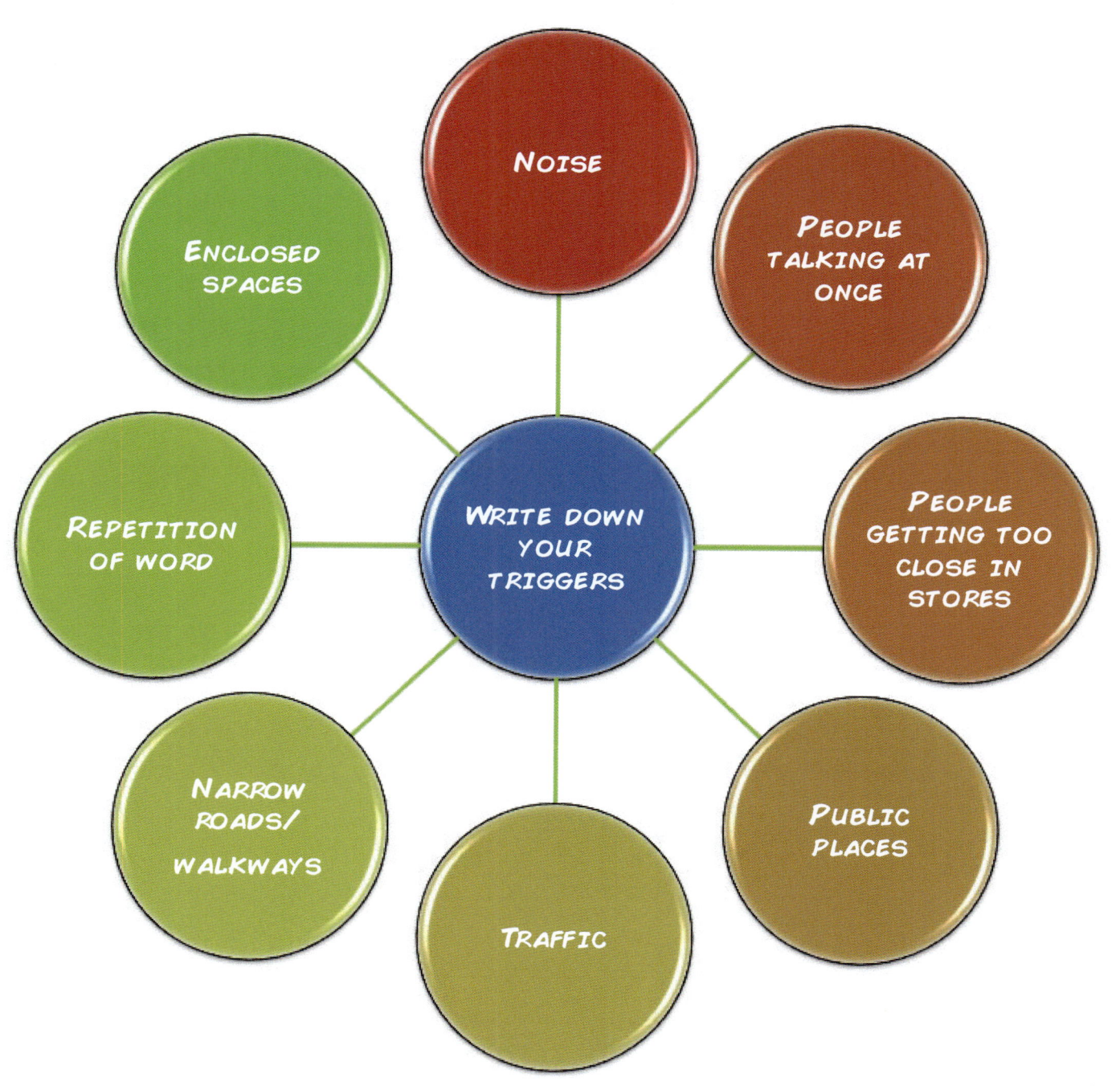

Write down your triggers

- Noise
- People talking at once
- People getting too close in stores
- Public places
- Traffic
- Narrow roads/walkways
- Repetition of word
- Enclosed spaces

Stay calm

The best thing to do is either

1. Remove ourselves from the trigger, or
2. Remove the trigger from ourselves

If this is not possible, try some of these...

Take a break

- Toilet cubicles
- Go outside
- Imagine somewhere relaxing

Calm your senses

- Noise reducing headphones
- Listen to relaxing music
- Put up hood
- Play with stress ball/toy
- Draw or colour a picture in a book

Allow others to help

- Stay with one person
- Ask them to arrange for you to get home
- Ask them to make an excuse for you
- Ask them to take over what you are doing

Plan in advance

- Routes/journeys
- Public transport connections
- Start/end times
- Monthly calendar view
- Do things early in the day

Make 'Traffic Light' Cards

It is not always easy to express how we are feeling, especially in times of high anxiety or stress. We can make our own coloured cards and show them to others when we start to feel anxious. The cards have a pre-agreed solution written on them, e.g.

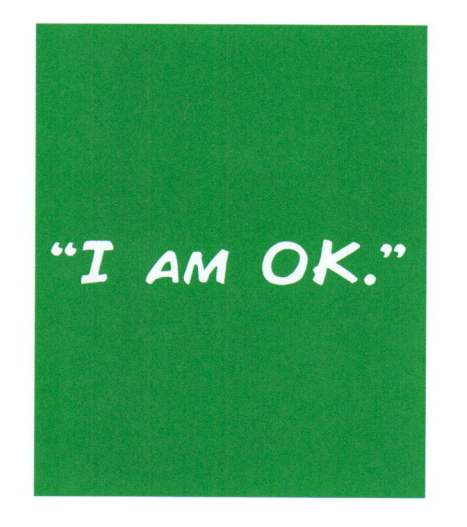

"I am OK."

1. "I need to find a person to talk to and ask for help
2. I need to use a calming method. E.g. Quiet space, music, headphones, etc."

"I am having a meltdown. I need my parent/guardian. Their contact details are..."

Use choices, not open-ends

If we don't know how to respond to something, it helps if the other person can provide a prompt by giving alternative options, e.g.

What would you like for lunch...

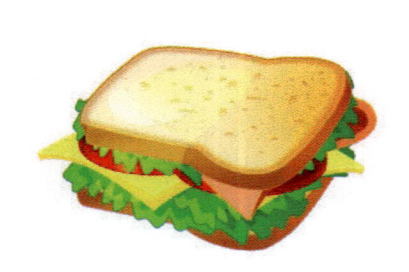

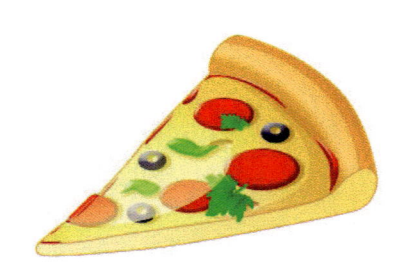

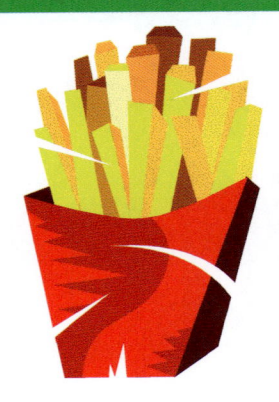

How would you like to travel...

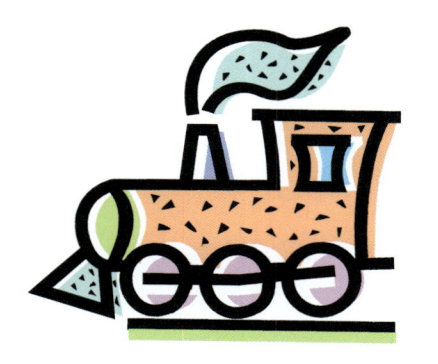

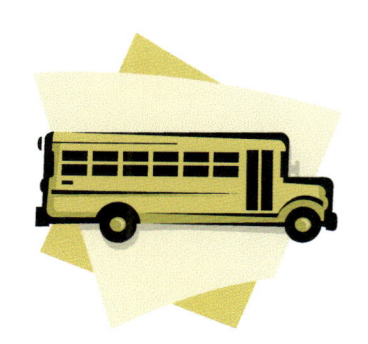

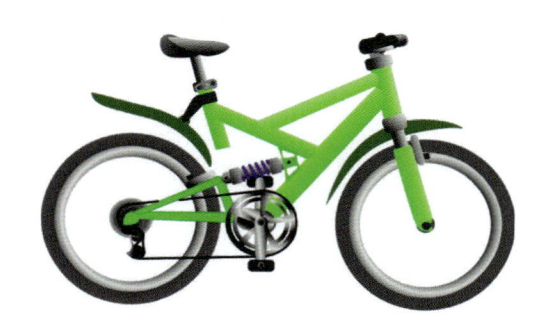

What would you like to do...

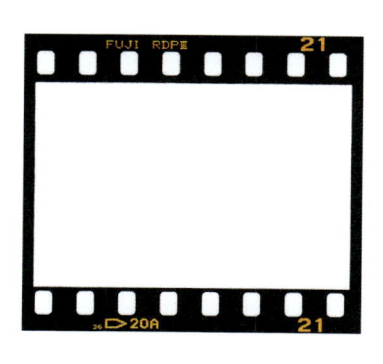

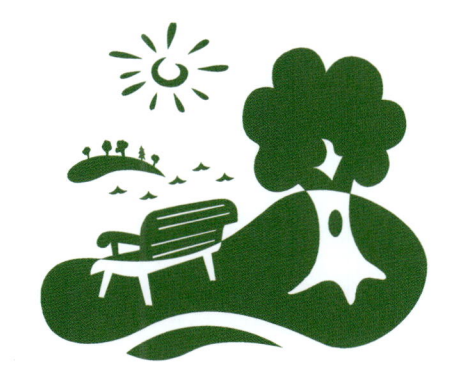

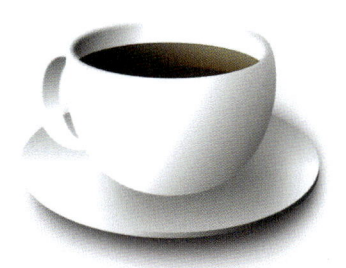

Strategies for anxiety in a social environment

Socialise Inside Structure

Social situations where there is a common/mutual goal are less anxiety-provoking

Structure	No structure
- Work - School - Board games - Reading club - Gym class - Cycling to a destination	- Party - Club/bar/pub - Coffee/tea - At friend's house

Declining invites

Always remember,
you do not have to say "yes"

Tell them as soon as you can

- It is polite to respond as soon as you can so they can make alternative arrangements
- If you can't make up your mind, just say "no"

Be clear

- Say "no" rather than "maybe" so as not to lead them on/give false hope
- Don't just not turn up

Give a reason (but you don't have to)

- "I have ASD and I find social situations very hard"
- "I have sensory processing issues and busy situations make me feel overwhelmed"
- It is OK to tell a white lie, such as "I am busy that day/evening" or "I'm not feeling well"

Thank them for the invite

- It is polite to thank them for thinking of you
- Let them know you are grateful to be asked
- Let them know to continue to ask you in the future, in case you one day change your mind

Don't feel bad about your decision

- It does not matter if you don't go to a party/social event
- Your well being comes first
- You are more likely to make others happy if you are happy
- "Fun" is relative – what one person finds fun, another may well find stressful

Take time to time-out

The space between the trigger and response is critical

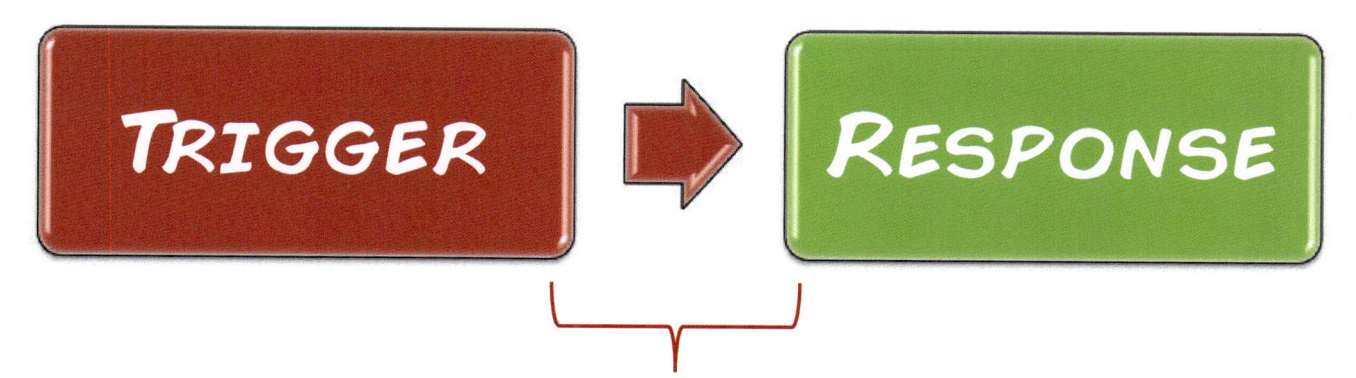

TRIGGER ➡ **RESPONSE**

Take time to timeout* inside this space

*Quietness, space, breathing, sensory indulgences, etc. Whatever your calming mechanisms are, use them

To finish...

You can only do your best

It's OK to be different

Respect what may be anxiety-provoking for you may be fun for somebody else, and vice versa

It's not worth putting yourself through so much anxiety and stress over things you really don't want to – or can't – do

Remind and reassure yourself that, even in the worst case scenario, you probably do have the skills to cope if things don't go to plan

Many thanks for reading

Other books in The Visual Guides series at the time of writing:

The Visual Guide to Asperger's Syndrome

The Visual Guide to Asperger's Syndrome Shutdowns and Meltdowns

The Visual Guide to Asperger's Syndrome in 5-8 Year Olds

The Visual Guide to Asperger's Syndrome in 8-11 Year Olds

The Visual Guide to Asperger's Syndrome in 13-16 Year Olds

The Visual Guide to Asperger's Syndrome for the Neurotypical Partner

New titles are continually being produced so keep an eye out!